YOU AND YOUR FERTILITY

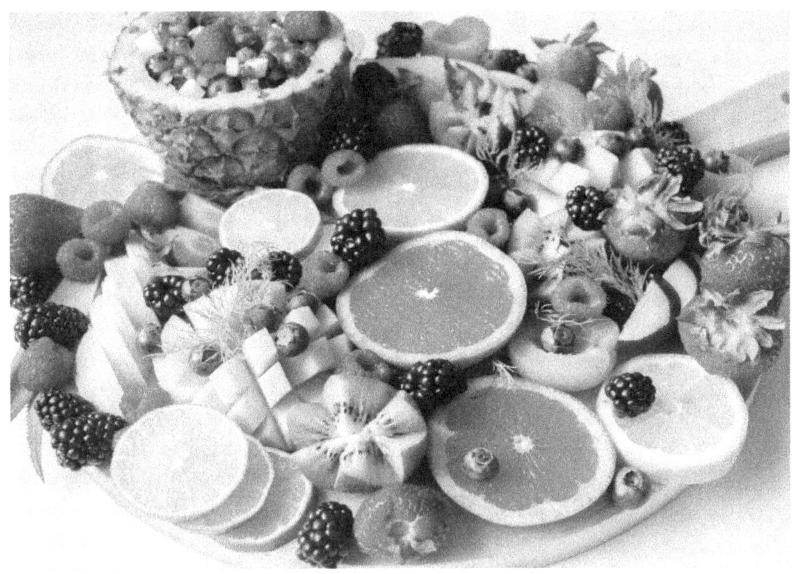

A simple guide to fertility,conception and pregnancy

By Lydia Sims

TABLE OF CONTENTS

	2
INTRODUCTION	5
CHAPTER ONE	**7**
UNDERSTANDING FERTILITY	7
Factors affecting fertility	9
Menstrual cycle and ovulation	10
Signs of fertility issues:	11
Preconception challenges	11
CHAPTER TWO	**14**
MANAGING FERTILITY ISSUES	14
Changes in Lifestyle	14
Medical Examination	16
CHAPTER THREE	**18**
Conception process	18
How conception occurs	18
1.Ovulation:	19
2. Fertilization:	19
3. ZygoteFormation:	19
4. Implantation:	19
5. Pregnancy Begins:	19
Common conception challenges	19
Importance of timing	20
CHAPTER FOUR	**22**
PREGNANCY	22
Confirming pregnancy	23
Stages of pregnancy	23
The second trimester(Weeks 13–16):	24
The third trimester (Weeks 29–40):	25
Gestational diabetes	26
Gestational hypertension	26
Important aspects of pregnancy	26
The Stages of Labor	27
Postpartum period:	28

CHAPTER FIVE   **30**

  MAKING THE PREGNANCY JOURNEY COMFORTABLE   30

    Health and Well-being   31

    Emotional well-being: 32

    Comfort   33

    Education and preparation: 33

  Choices of giving birth   33

  Conclusion   35

INTRODUCTION

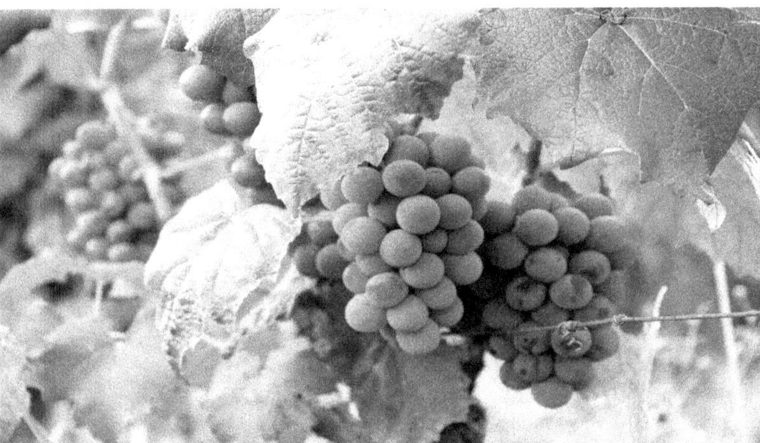

In a quaint countryside nestled between rolling hills and fertile fields,At the heart of this village lived Maya, a young woman whose heart resonated with the desire for a family. Surrounded by the lush bounty of nature, Maya was raised with the wisdom passed down through generations,the understanding that the earth's gifts held the key to vitality and fertility.From the golden kernels of corn to the vibrant hues of assorted fruits and vegetables, the villagers believed that the bounty of the land was more than sustenance,it was a pathway to vitality and the promise of fertility. Maya, inspired by this belief, tended to the family garden with utmost care, nurturing a variety of nutrient-rich plants, fruits, and vegetables that adorned their home.With each passing season,Maya diligently cultivated a diverse array of produce;leafy greens, colorful peppers,succulent fruits, and an assortment of herbs renowned for their healthful properties. The family's meals were a canvas painted with the vibrant hues and flavors of the earth's bounty,a celebration of life's nourishment from nature's cornucopia.

As Maya savored each wholesome bite, she embraced the belief that the goodness harvested from the land would infuse her body with vitality, creating an optimal environment for the fulfillment of her aspirations for motherhood.Days turned into months, and Maya's devotion to

the garden and its nutritious offerings continued unwaveringly. She found solace and purpose in nurturing the plants, understanding that their vitality mirrored her own.One serene evening, as the village basked in the warm glow of the setting sun, Maya's heart skipped a beat, a moment of realization dawned upon her. Nestled among the verdant rows of her beloved garden, she felt an inexplicable sense of gratitude and connection. Her journey toward fertility was not just about consuming the bounty of the land but embracing the harmony and life force pulsating within it. Months passed, and the garden flourished under Maya's tender care. Mirroring the vibrant bloom of her family's garden, Maya's life took a new turn,a blossom of hope and joy as she discovered she was carrying a life within her, a testament to the nourishment and vitality bestowed upon her by the land's abundant blessings.

CHAPTER ONE

UNDERSTANDING FERTILITY

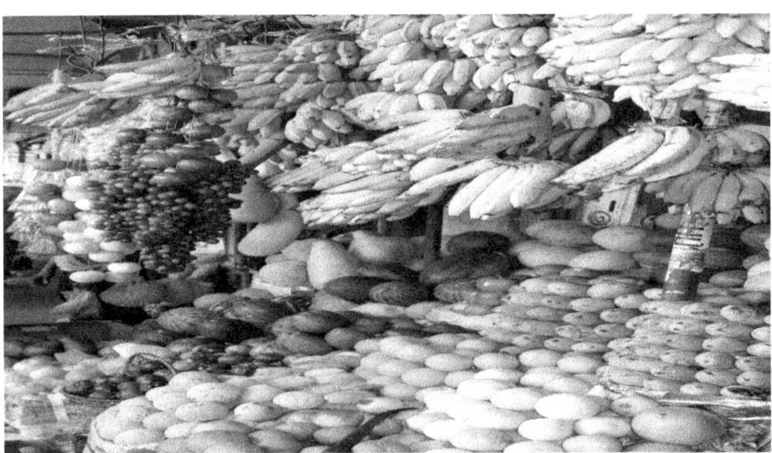

In human terms, it refers to the ability of an individual, either male or female, to contribute to conception and facilitate the birth of a child.
Female fertility involves a complex interplay of physiological, hormonal, and reproductive factors. Understanding the key components of female fertility can aid in comprehending how various factors influence a woman's ability to conceive:

Ovarian Reserve: This refers to a woman's remaining egg supply. A woman is born with a certain number of eggs, and this supply decreases with age. Ovarian reserve gives an indication of the quantity and quality of the eggs remaining in the ovaries. Diminished ovarian reserve can impact fertility and decrease the chances of conception.

Hormonal Balance: Hormones play a crucial role in regulating the menstrual cycle and supporting fertility. Hormones such as follicle-stimulating hormone (FSH), luteinizing hormone (LH), estrogen, and progesterone are involved in the process of ovulation and the preparation of the uterus for pregnancy. Any disruptions in hormonal balance can affect ovulation and fertility.

Factors affecting fertility

Fertility, or the ability to conceive and bring a pregnancy to term, is affected by a variety of factors, including biological, environmental, lifestyle, and health-related factors. Here are some important factors influencing fertility:

Age: Both men and women's fertility are affected by their age. Women's fertility declines as they age, owing to a decrease in the amount and quality of eggs. Men, like women, endure a steady loss in fertility, but at a slower rate.

Reproductive Health: Fertility depends on both male and female reproductive health. Polycystic ovarian syndrome (PCOS), endometriosis, fibroids, sexually transmitted infections (STIs), and anatomical abnormalities in either partner can all have an impact on fertility.

The frequency and timing of sexual intercourse can have an impact on fertility. Understanding the menstrual cycle and engaging in sexual activity during the woman's viable window (around ovulation) increases the likelihood of conception.

Genetic Factors: Fertility can be influenced by genetic factors. Some genetic diseases can impact both men and women's reproductive health, resulting in infertility.

Obesity and underweight: both have an impact on fertility. Obesity can affect hormone levels and ovulation in women, while it can contribute to poor sperm quality and erectile dysfunction in males. Being underweight can also impact hormone levels in both sexes, causing menstrual cycle irregularities and decreased sperm production in males.

Environmental factors: Exposure to some environmental factors, such as pesticides, chemicals, pollutants, and radiation, may have an effect on both male and female fertility.

Medical Conditions and therapies: Diabetes, thyroid disorders, autoimmune diseases, and cancer therapies such as chemotherapy or radiation can all have an affect on fertility. Medications used to treat a variety of medical issues may have an impact on fertility. Understanding these factors and their possible impact on fertility might help people take proactive measures to improve their reproductive health. Seeking medical assistance from a healthcare practitioner is critical, especially if you are suffering fertility issues. Fertility specialists can offer advice, do fertility tests, and propose appropriate therapies or lifestyle modifications to increase the odds of conception.

Menstrual cycle and ovulation

Menstrual cycle: The menstrual cycle is a crucial aspect of female fertility. It typically lasts about 28 days but can vary widely among individuals. Ovulation, the release of a mature egg from the ovary, usually occurs around the midpoint of the cycle. The egg is available for fertilization for about 12-24 hours after ovulation.
An important stage of a woman's menstrual cycle is ovulation, which usually happens in the middle of the cycle. It is the procedure via which an egg reaches maturity, breaks off from the ovary, and becomes ready for fertilization. The pituitary gland produces both luteinizing hormone (LH) and follicle-stimulating hormone (FSH), which play a major role in the intricate interaction of hormones that regulate ovulation.
Ovulation:an important stage of a woman's menstrual cycle is ovulation, which usually happens in the middle of the cycle. It is the procedure via which an egg reaches maturity, breaks off from Í ovary, and becomes ready for fertilization. The pituitary gland produces both luteinizing Iphormone (LH) and follicle-stimulating hormone (FSH), which play a major role in the intricate interaction of hormones that regulate ovulation.
The luteal phase and the follicular phase are the two main phases of the menstrual cycle. Menstruation marks the start of the follicular phase, when FSH promotes the growth of ovarian follicles, each of which contains an immature egg. These follicles produce estrogen as they develop, which causes the uterine lining to alter in anticipation of a possible pregnancy.A rise in LH happens as the follicular phase develops; this usually happens around day 14 of a typical 28-day cycle. Ovulation begins when this rise in LH causes the mature egg to be released from the follicle. After being discharged, the egg passes through the fallopian tube and may fertilize when it comes into contact with sperm.

For those attempting to conceive or avoid getting pregnant, it is essential to understand their menstrual cycle. Ovulation can be predicted by a number of techniques, including monitoring basal body temperature, monitoring changes in cervical mucus, and using ovulation predictor kits. In addition, women may notice a slight increase in their sense of smell or moderate pelvic

pain during ovulation.The fragments of the burst follicle that remain become the corpus luteum if fertilization is unsuccessful.

Progesterone, which is produced by the corpus luteum, aids in maintaining the uterine lining throughout pregnancy. The corpus luteum degenerates and the cycle restarts in the absence of pregnancy.

Signs of fertility issues:

Irregular menstrual cycle: Ovulatory issues may be the cause of irregular or nonexistent menstrual cycles.

Menstrual discomfort: Severe cramping during the menstrual cycle or pelvic pain may indicate endometriosis or other related disorders.

Hormonal imbalance: Disorders like PCOS, or polycystic ovarian syndrome, can cause hormonal imbalances that have an impact on fertility.

Age related factor: Women over 35 may have difficulty conceiving, and fertility decreases with age.

Prior miscarriages: A history of many miscarriages may indicate underlying problems with reproduction.

Before attempting to conceive, individuals or couples might undertake a preconception health check-up, which consists of a medical evaluation and counseling session. In order to increase the likelihood of a successful pregnancy and advance the health of the unborn child as well as the prospective parents, this proactive step is intended to evaluate and optimize a number of health factors.

In the course of a preconception health examination, medical practitioners usually address:

Preconception challenges

1. Health background:

Examine your medical history thoroughly, as well as that of your family, to rule out any genetic or inherited disorders that could affect the pregnancy.

Recognise prior reproductive experiences, such as any problems, miscarriages, or conceptions.

2. **Vaccinations**:
 Make sure that both partners have received the most recent shots to protect against infectious diseases that could be dangerous during pregnancy.
Talk about any additional vaccinations, such the flu shot, that are advised for expectant mothers.
3. **Infection Screening**:

Perform thorough screening for sexually transmitted infections (STIs) in order to identify and treat any illnesses that may compromise fertility or endanger the developing fetus.
Take into account getting tested for additional infections that may affect pregnancy, such as hepatitis and rubella.
4. **Nutritional Assessment**:
Assess eating patterns to make sure they are nutrient-dense, highlighting the significance of calcium, iron, folic acid, and other important vitamins and minerals.
Talk about the possibility of utilizing dietary supplements and create a food plan that is well-balanced.
5. **Lifestyle factors**:
Talk about lifestyle choices such drinking alcohol, smoking cigarettes, and using drugs; stress the need of cutting back or using them sparingly in order to maximize[7] fertility and pregnancy outcomes.
Promote regular exercise and stress reduction as essential elements of reproductive health.
6.**Weight Management**:
Since being underweight or overweight might affect fertility and pregnancy, it is important to evaluate body weight and body mass index (BMI) to see if any changes are necessary.
Create a customized plan for changing your lifestyle to reach and maintain a healthy weight.
7. **Chronic issues**:
To reduce risks during pregnancy, manage and stabilize chronic health issues such as diabetes, hypertension, or thyroid disorders before becoming pregnant.
Work collaboratively with medical professionals to maximize the administration of medications for long-term diseases.
8.**Medication reviews**:
Make sure all over-the-counter and prescription drugs are safe to take during pregnancy by reviewing them.
If necessary, change the dosage of your medications, and look into less risky solutions for the growing fetus.
9. **Reproductive Health**:
Assess menstrual cycles and take care of any anomalies or issues that can affect a woman's ability to conceive.

Address any past medical history of reproductive problems, such as endometriosis or polycystic ovarian syndrome (PCOS), and carry out the necessary treatments.

10. **Guidance**:

Provide thorough preconception counseling, including issues with diet, exercise, emotional health, and prenatal care.

Address any particular worries or inquiries that the individuals or couples may have about getting pregnant and being pregnant.

During preconception health check-ups, having candid and in-depth conversations with medical professionals guarantees a comprehensive approach to optimizing fertility and fostering a safe pregnancy.

CHAPTER TWO

MANAGING FERTILITY ISSUES

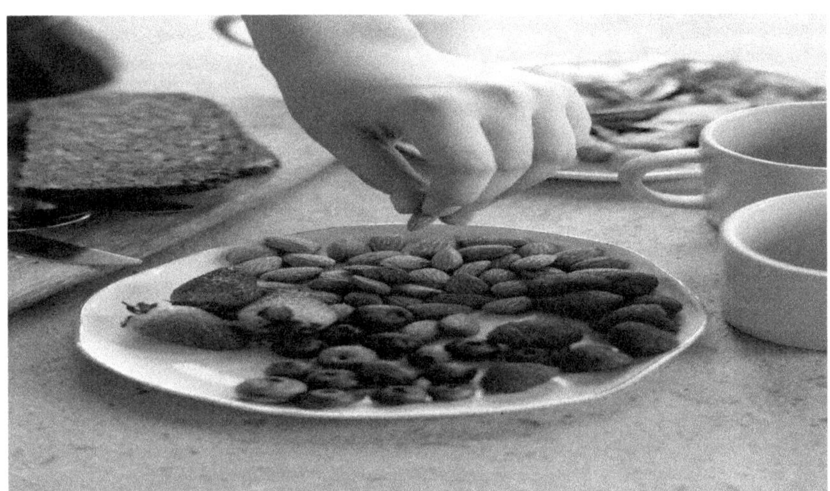

Managing fertility issues necessitates a holistic strategy that includes medical, behavioral, emotional, and supportive factors. Here's a thorough rundown:

Changes in Lifestyle

●Dietary Guidelines: Eating a well-balanced diet high in nutrients, vitamins, and antioxidants can help with fertility. It is beneficial to consume foods that promote hormonal balance and reproductive wellness.Several fruits and vegetables have nutritional qualities that may aid fertility by delivering important vitamins, minerals, antioxidants, and other nutrients. While there is no certainty that eating these foods will result in conception, combining them into a healthy diet may improve reproductive health. Here are some foods and vegetables that are frequently recommended to help with fertility:

1. Dark Leafy Greens: Spinach, Kale and Swiss Chard are high in folate, a B vitamin that may help with ovulation and pregnancy health.

Blueberries, raspberries, and strawberries are abundant in antioxidants, notably vitamin C and flavonoids, which may help minimize oxidative stress and increase egg quality.

3. Citrus Fruits: Oranges, Lemons, Grapefruits: Citrus fruits are high in vitamin C, which aids male and female fertility by boosting sperm health and hormone balance.

4. Avocado: Avocados are high in monounsaturated fats, which are necessary for hormone production and may help in ovulation.

5. Cruciferous veggies: Broccoli, Cauliflower, Brussels Sprouts: These veggies contain folate, vitamins, and minerals that maintain hormonal balance and may aid in fertility improvement.

Sweet potatoes are high in beta-carotene and a strong source of vitamin A, which is important for reproductive health and may aid healthy fetal development.

Pomegranates: Pomegranate seeds are abundant in antioxidants and have been linked to enhanced sperm quality.

8. Bananas: Bananas are high in vitamin B6, which may help regulate hormones and promote fertility.

9. Asparagus: Asparagus is high in folate and other nutrients that promote reproductive health and may aid in conception.

Tomatoes include lycopene, an antioxidant that has been shown to improve sperm quality and motility in males.

Consuming a variety of colorful fruits and vegetables as part of a well-balanced and nutritious diet can supply a wide range of critical elements that support overall health, including reproductive health. While these foods may help with fertility, it's vital to work with a healthcare practitioner or a certified dietitian for personalised dietary suggestions that are customised to individual health needs and any unique fertility difficulties.

•Regular physical activity aids in weight maintenance and may boost fertility.Excessive exercise, on the other hand, can occasionally have a detrimental impact on fertility, so moderation is essential.

•Avoiding Harmful Substances: It is critical to limit or avoid alcohol, smoking, recreational drugs, and exposure to environmental toxins or pollution.

Medical Examination

1.Fertility Evaluation: To identify any issues, both partners should undergo a comprehensive fertility evaluation. Physical examinations, blood tests, sperm analysis for men, imaging studies, and menstrual cycle assessments for women are all routine.

Finding the Root Causes: Identifying and treating underlying illnesses such as hormone imbalances, polycystic ovarian syndrome (PCOS), endometriosis, fibroids, or structural issues can significantly improve reproductive prospects.

2.Fertility medicines: Hormonal medicines can increase ovulation in women and improve sperm production in men.

Intrauterine Insemination (IUI): To boost the chances of fertilization, prepared sperm is placed directly into the uterus around the time of ovulation.

IVF (In Vitro Fertilisation): IVF is the process of fertilizing eggs with sperm outside of the body and then implanting the resulting embryo(s) into the uterus.

Intracytoplasmic Sperm Injection (ICSI): This procedure, performed in conjunction with IVF, involves injecting a single sperm directly into an egg to help with fertilization.

3.Surgery: Surgical operations may be required to correct fertility-related anatomical abnormalities such as obstructed fallopian tubes, fibroids, or endometrial polyps.

4. Assisted Reproductive Technologies (ART): ART includes modern techniques for conception such as IVF, ICSI, egg or sperm donation, and embryo freezing (cryopreservation), among others.

5. Emotional Support and Counseling: Fertility concerns can be emotionally difficult. Counselors, support groups, or therapists that specialize in fertility-related issues can help individuals and couples manage the emotional aspects.

6.Alternative Therapies, including acupuncture, herbal supplements, meditation, and yoga, can help with fertility. While not scientifically validated as stand-alone treatments, they may supplement traditional reproductive treatments.

Navigating reproductive challenges frequently necessitates a personalized approach that is suited to each individual or couple's unique requirements and circumstances. Consulting with fertility specialists, reproductive endocrinologists, or infertility specialists can give personalized treatment regimens and ongoing support throughout the fertility process. Furthermore, maintaining open communication, finding emotional support, and being informed about available options are critical components of fertility management.

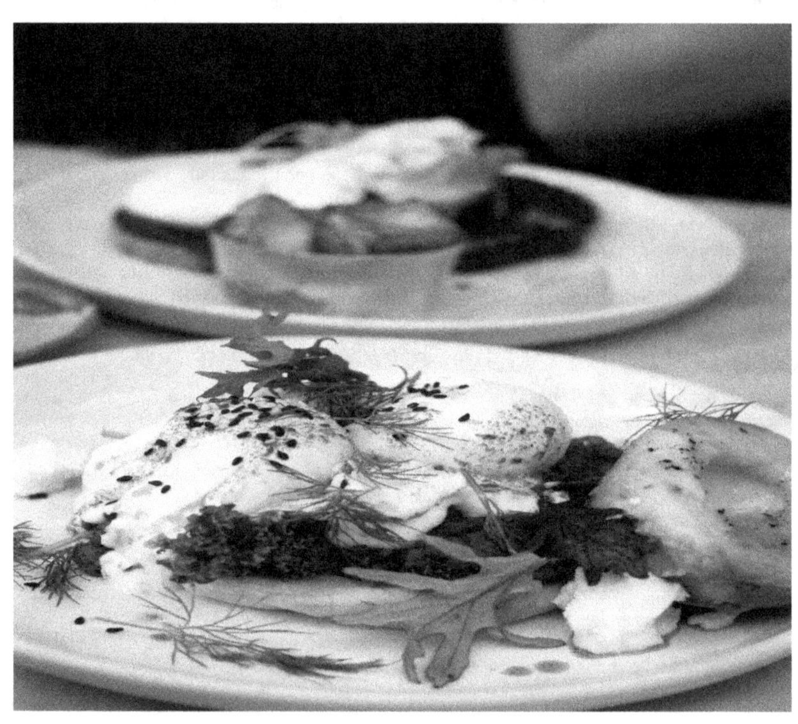

CHAPTER THREE

Conception process

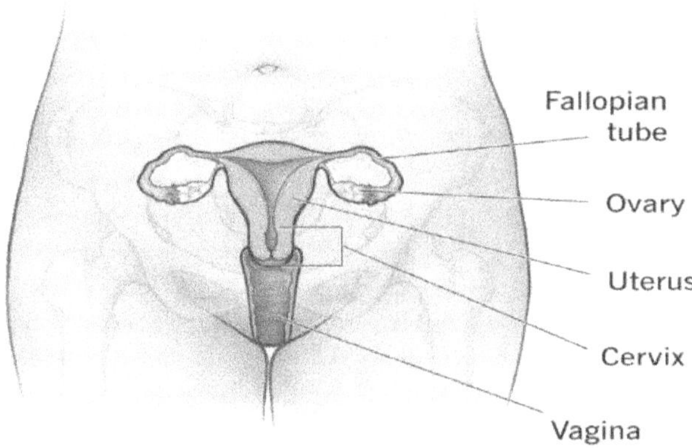

How conception occurs

Conception is the first step of pregnancy, where a sperm cell fertilizes an egg, culminating in the development of a zygote. It is a critical biological event that signals the start of a new life. This is a complete summary of the conceptualization process.

1.Ovulation:

The release of a mature egg from one of the ovaries is the first step in the process of conception. Ovulation occurs when a woman's luteinizing hormone (LH) levels rise, usually around the midway of her menstrual cycle. The egg is then liberated from the ovary and enters the fallopian tube.

2. Fertilization:

Sexual intercourse during the fertile window, which is often around the time of ovulation, permits sperm to enter the female reproductive system. Sperm can live in the female reproductive system for several days expecting the release of an egg.
When a sperm cell penetrates and fertilizes an egg in the fallopian tube, it generates a zygote. The fusing of genetic material from the sperm and egg results in the formation of a new single-celled organism, which initiates cell division and embryonic development.

3. ZygoteFormation:

 The zygote divides rapidly, resulting in a cluster of cells known as a blastocyst. This stage of development happens as the blastocyst moves via the fallopian tube and into the uterus.

4. Implantation:

About 6-10 days after fertilization, the blastocyst enters the uterus. It connects to the uterine lining (endometrium) during implantation. Once implanted, the blastocyst continues to develop and grow.

5. Pregnancy Begins:

 Pregnancy begins when the blastocyst effectively implants in the uterine lining. Hormonal changes occur, directing the body to assist the developing embryo and prepare for pregnancy.

Common conception challenges

1.Timing and Ovulation: Having intercourse during the fertile window surrounding ovulation enhances the likelihood of conception.

2.Sperm Health: Sperm quality, count, and motility are critical components of effective fertilization.

3.Egg Health: The health and viability of the egg play an important part in conception.

4.Reproductive Health: Conditions affecting the reproductive organs, hormone imbalances, or structural difficulties can all have an impact on conception.

5.Age: Both male and female fertility decrease with age, reducing the chances of conception. Conception is a complex biological process affected by a variety of circumstances. While it happens naturally in many circumstances, certain people or couples may have difficulty conceiving because of reproductive concerns. Seeking medical guidance and assistance from healthcare specialists, especially if conception issues persist, can aid in recognising and overcoming potential barriers to pregnancy.

Importance of timing

For several reasons, the timing of conception is important. First of all, a woman's fertility is cyclical; by recognising the menstrual cycle, one may determine the optimal window for conception, improving the odds of a successful pregnancy. Furthermore, the best time guarantees a healthy environment for the embryo, lowering the possibility of issues. Furthermore, a woman's lifestyle, stress levels, and general health can all influence the success of her conception. All things considered, a well-timed pregnancy increases the chances of success and health.

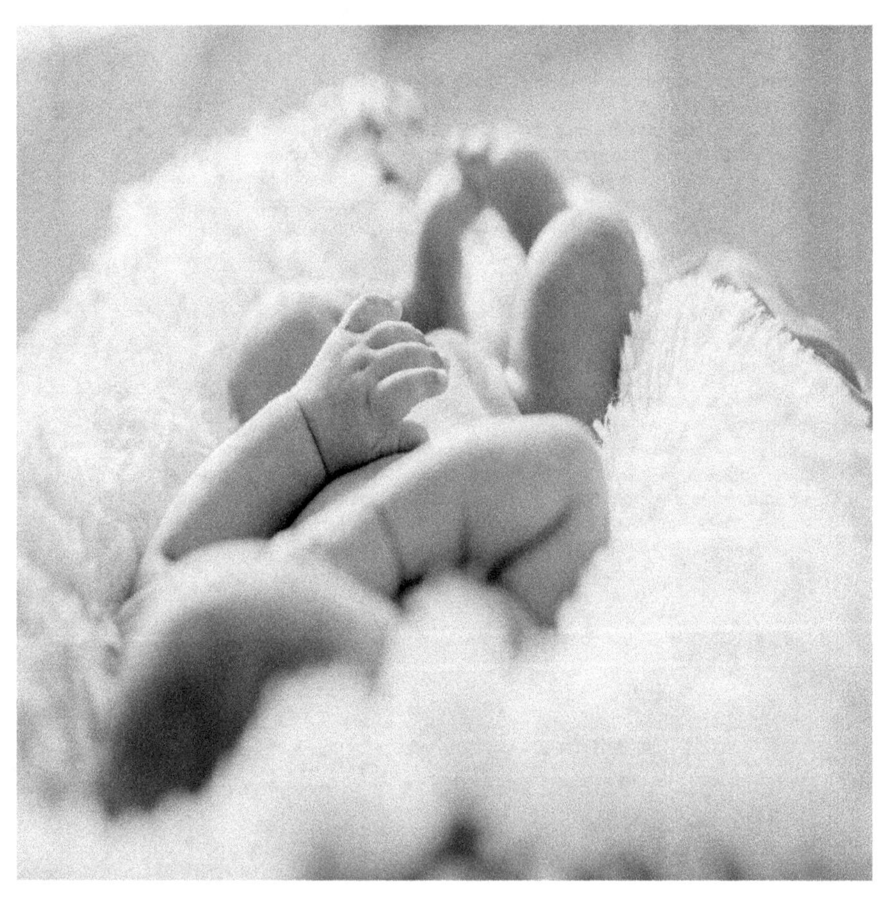

CHAPTER FOUR

PREGNANCY

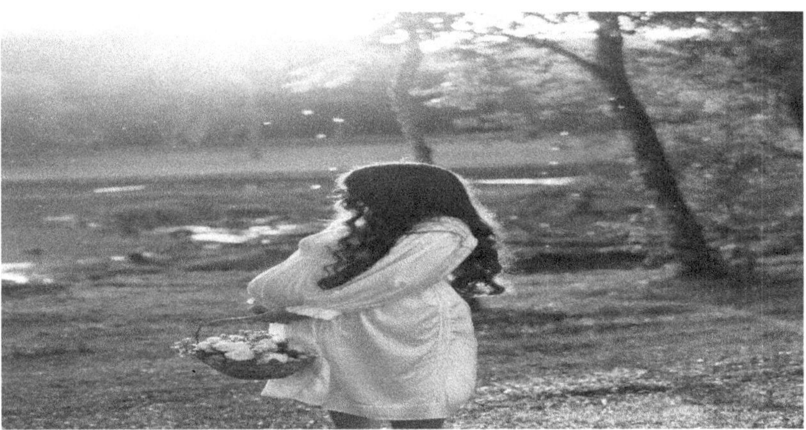

 Pregnancy is a transformational and intricate process in which a fertilized egg develops into a fetus, finally giving birth to a baby. It is separated into three trimesters, each lasting around three months and causing major changes in a woman's body to support the growing fetus. Here's a complete overview of pregnancy.

Confirming pregnancy

Taking a home pregnancy test, which is available at pharmacies, or getting a blood test from a healthcare professional are the usual methods for confirming pregnancy. The hormone called

hCG, which is created during pregnancy, is detected by both techniques. Seeking advice from a healthcare expert guarantees precise outcomes and direction for further actions.

Stages of pregnancy

The first trimester of pregnancy,which lasts from week 1 to week 12, is a critical time for the development of the embryo. These significant junctures occur during this stage:
Weeks 1-4: Implantation and Conception
Usually, fertilization happens in week two.
By week four, a ball of cells called a blastocyst forms and implants into the uterine lining.
Week 5: Development of Neural Tubes
The neural tube starts to form, eventually developing into the brain and spinal cord.
The heart begins to beat at a basic level.
Week 6: Limb buds and heartbeat
The heart begins to form its chambers and beats audibly.
When limb buds first appear, arm and leg creation is just getting started.
Week 8: Development of Organs
The formation of major organs such as the kidneys, liver, and lungs begins.Eyes and ears among other facial features become identifiable.
Week Ten: Female Genitalia
Sexual distinction emerges, even though an ultrasound might not show it.
The baby is called a fetus when its webbed fingers and toes separate.
Week 12: Motions of the Fetus
The mother usually does not feel the fetal movements at first.
The fetus is roughly the size of a lime and has all major organ systems in place.

Expectant mothers may have symptoms such as exhaustion, mood fluctuations, and morning sickness, which is common in the first trimester of pregnancy, can be difficult to deal with, but there are a few techniques to help:

Smaller, More Often Meals: Try eating smaller, more frequent meals throughout the day as an alternative to three large ones. By doing so, you can avoid having an empty stomach, which can exacerbate nausea, and help stabilize blood sugar levels.

Remain Hydrated: It's important to maintain adequate fluids because dehydration can make nausea worse. Drink water throughout the day and think about flavoring it with a slice of lemon to aid with nausea.

Avoid Triggers: Recognise and steer clear of foods or odors that make you feel queasy. Morning sickness can occasionally get worse when around strong smells, such those of cooking or perfume.

Ginger: The anti-nausea effects of ginger have long been recognised. You may attempt Ginger sweets, tea, and supplements are all options. Be sure to speak with your doctor before taking any supplements while expecting.

Food Cravings and Aversions: In spite of aversions, strive for a balanced diet.In moderation, give in to urges.
Mood swings: Talk to your support network and spouse.Take part in relaxing and uplifting activities.
Constipation: Eat a diet high in dietary fibre.Continue your physical activity.
Headaches: Drink plenty of water.Use calming strategies.
For specific guidance, always speak with your healthcare practitioner. If symptoms are severe or persistent, consult a physician right once.
During the first trimester. Frequent prenatal exams, such as ultrasound scans, assist keep an eye on the developing baby and guarantee the mother's health. Additionally, this is a critical period for genetic testing and potential problem screening.

The second trimester(Weeks 13–16):

Physical Changes: Weariness and nausea may lessen. The features on the baby's face grow.

Fetal Development: The infant begins to produce urine as its organs continue to form.
Emotional Aspects: Feeling better and having more energy are possible outcomes of alleviating early pregnancy discomfort.
Weeks 17–20: Physical Changes: A more visible baby bump appears. An ultrasound can be used to determine gender.
Fetal Development: The mother feels the quickening of the baby's movements. The baby's body is covered in fine hair, or lanugo.
Emotional aspects: As the baby's movements become more noticeable, your bond with them gets stronger.
Physical Changes: Weight Gain Continues in Weeks 21–24. There may be symptoms of stretching in the mother's skin.
Fetal Development: The lungs continue to mature while the baby's sense organs grow.

Emotional Aspects: As a kid becomes more viable outside the womb, feelings of assurance and confidence frequently grow.

Weeks 25–28: A shift in the body Some moms get leg cramps and a sore back. There may be variations in blood pressure.
Fetal Development: The infant's eyes open, and its brain begins to do increasingly complex tasks.
Emotional Aspects: Talks about parenting and birthing plans may get more intense as part of the prenatal preparations.

The third trimester (Weeks 29–40):

Physical Changes: Getting uncomfortable because the baby is growing. Contractions from Braxton Hicks may start to show.
Fetal Development: The infant puts on a lot of weight and its bones get harder.
Emotional Aspects: As the deadline draws near, feelings of anticipation and even apprehension may surface.
Weeks 33–36: Physical Changes: The position of the baby is tracked in preparation for delivery. There could be hand and foot swelling.
Fetal Development: The infant develops breathing techniques and fortifies its defenses against infection.
Emotional Aspects: Nesting impulses could take over and make plans for the baby's arrival necessary.
Physical changes occur in weeks 37–40 when the baby lowers into the pelvis in preparation for birth. There could be a mucus plug discharge.

Fetal Development: The baby's immune system is ready, and its organs are fully developed.
Emotional Aspects: As the due date draws closer, there will likely be a range of feelings experienced. Increased attention is paid to labor indicators.
The start of labor and subsequent delivery mark the end of the third trimester.

Gestational diabetes

One kind of diabetes that appears during pregnancy is called gestational diabetes. It alters the way your body metabolizes sugar, which raises blood sugar levels. It may raise the possibility of difficulties developing during pregnancy and childbirth. Gestational diabetes is commonly managed with blood sugar monitoring, a nutritious diet, and occasionally medication. It usually goes away after childbirth, but it raises the chance of type 2 diabetes in later life.

Gestational hypertension

Gestational hypertension, or elevated blood pressure during pregnancy, can be dangerous for both the mother and the unborn child. Preeclampsia, a more serious illness marked by elevated blood pressure and damage to vital organs including the liver and kidneys, is one of the problems that could arise from it. Preeclampsia can impact placenta function, which may result in very low birth weight or early birth.

Managing high blood pressure during pregnancy requires regular blood pressure checks, adherence to medical instructions, and a healthy lifestyle. In severe circumstances, medication or an early birth may be necessary to avoid difficulties. For the purpose of monitoring and controlling blood pressure during pregnancy, routine prenatal care and communication with healthcare practitioners are essential.

Important aspects of pregnancy

1. **Prenatal Care**. Regular prenatal check-ups with healthcare experts are essential throughout the pregnancy. These appointments include evaluating the mother's health and the baby's growth, as well as treating any concerns or difficulties that may occur.

2.**Healthy Lifestyle**: A healthy pregnancy includes eating a balanced diet, being physically active (with a healthcare provider's consent), taking prenatal vitamins, avoiding dangerous drugs (such as alcohol, tobacco, and certain medications), and managing stress.

3.**Labor and Delivery**: Typically, labor begins when contractions become regular and the cervix dilates.

The Stages of Labor

- First Stage (Dilation): Early Labor:

Contractions begin, and the cervix starts to efface (thin out) and dilate (open). Contractions may be irregular and mild initially. Active Labor: Contractions become more intense and regular, and the cervix continues to dilate. This is a more challenging phase for the mother, often requiring focus and coping strategies. Transitional Labor: The final phase of the first stage where the

cervix reaches full dilation (10 centimeters). Contractions are strong and close together. Some women experience intense emotions and physical sensations during this phase.

- Second Stage (Pushing and Delivery):

Begins when the cervix is fully dilated, and the woman feels an urge to push. This stage involves active pushing to propel the baby through the birth canal. The baby's head emerges first, followed by the shoulders and the rest of the body. The birth of the baby concludes this stage.

- Third Stage (Placental Delivery):

After the baby is born, the uterus continues to contract, causing the placenta to separate from the uterine wall. The placenta is expelled through the birth canal, usually within 5-30 minutes after the baby's birth. Some healthcare providers may facilitate this process by gently pulling on the umbilical cord or administering medications to aid in placental delivery. These stages collectively represent the natural progression of childbirth. However, it's crucial to recognize that labor experiences can vary, and interventions or complications may necessitate adjustments to this typical pattern.

Postpartum period:

After birth, the postpartum period includes the mother's healing, bonding with the newborn, and adjusting to the new family dynamic. As the mother's body recovers from pregnancy, she experiences physical and emotional changes.

Postpartum care:

1. Physical Recuperation: Health Monitoring To monitor the mother's physical recovery and take immediate action in the event of any difficulties, routine check-ups are crucial.

Nutrition: Both nursing and postpartum recuperation depend on a well-balanced diet. Drinking enough water is also essential.

Exercise: Rebuilding strength and endurance can be facilitated by introducing mild workouts gradually.

2. Emotional Assistance: Awareness of Postpartum Depression: It's critical to recognise the symptoms of postpartum depression. Family and friend support on an emotional level is crucial, as is seeking professional assistance when necessary.

Bonding: Promoting a strong link between a mother and her infant helps them both feel emotionally healthy.

3. Support for nursing: Lactation Consultation: Advice from lactation consultants can help with difficulties related to nursing.

Nutritional Support: A mother's ability to successfully nurse her child depends on her diet.

4. Sleep and Rest: Getting Enough Sleep: Making sure the mother getting enough sleep is essential for the mother's healing. Tasks around the house can be helped by friends and family.

5. Contraception and Family Planning: As part of postpartum care, families should talk about and make plans for future pregnancies. Selecting an effective method of contraception is crucial.

6. Keeping an Eye on and Handling Complications:

Prevention of Infections: Infections at the site of delivery or in the incisions made during a C-section can be avoided with good cleaning and care.

Handling Postpartum Haemorrhage: It's critical to identify and treat any severe bleeding as soon as possible.

7. Postpartum Check-ups: Frequent Aftercare: Regular postpartum check-ups with medical professionals guarantee that the mother's and the child's health are regularly checked.

8. Support System: Social Support: A mother's emotional health can be greatly enhanced by having a solid support network that consists of her spouse, family, and friends.

9 Exercises for the Pelvic Floor These exercises support bladder control, promote overall healing, and strengthen the pelvic muscles.

10. Considering Mental Health:
Therapeutic Support: Getting help for stress, anxiety, or other mental health issues may benefit from counseling or therapy, if necessary.

The goal of comprehensive postpartum care is to satisfy the mother's physical, emotional, and practical needs during this critical time by working together with her support system and healthcare providers. Having regular awareness and communication helps the postpartum period go more smoothly.
Pregnancy is a unique and transforming experience that causes profound physical, emotional, and psychological changes. Each pregnancy is unique, and while it is a natural process, getting proper medical care, guidance, and support is critical for a successful pregnancy.

CHAPTER FIVE

MAKING THE PREGNANCY JOURNEY COMFORTABLE

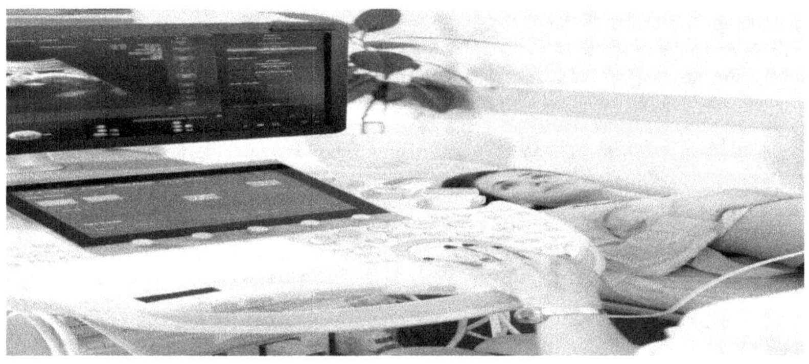

While it may provide problems, there are several ways to make the journey easier and more comfortable. Here are some extensive tips:

Health and Well-being

1.Regular Prenatal Care: Schedule regular check-ups with your healthcare practitioner. These sessions assist to monitor the mother's and baby's health and ensure that any difficulties are handled as soon as possible.

2.Balanced Nutrition: Consume a varied diet rich in fruits, vegetables, lean proteins, whole grains, and dairy.Here's a comprehensive list of foods, vegetables, and dairy products that are good for pregnant women:

Fruits:

1.Bananas are high in potassium, which helps to regulate blood pressure.
2.Oranges: Oranges are high in Vitamin C, which aids in iron absorption and boosts immunity.
3.Avocados are high in healthy fats, folate, and potassium, making them excellent for fetal development.

4.Berries (strawberries, blueberries, and raspberries): Berries are high in antioxidants and vitamins, making them beneficial to general health.
5.Apples are high in fiber and vital nutrients, which improve digestive health.

Vegetables:
1.Leafy greens (spinach, kale and Swiss chard): These greens are high in folate, iron, and fiber, making them crucial for fetal development.
2.Sweet potatoes are high in Vitamin A, which helps the baby's growth and development.
Broccoli: Packed with calcium, folate, and fiber, broccoli promotes bone health and digestion.
3.Bell peppers are high in vitamin C and antioxidants, which help to improve the immune system.
4.Carrots are high in beta-carotene, which promotes eye and skin health.

Dairy:
1.Milk: Milk, which is high in calcium and protein, helps babies develop their bones and muscles.
2.Greek Yogurt: High in probiotics, protein, and calcium, Greek yogurt promotes digestion and bone health.
3.Cheese is high in calcium and protein, which promotes bone formation.
Fortified Plant-Based Milks (Almond Milk, Soy Milk): These plant-based milks are fortified with calcium and vitamin D, which are beneficial to bone health.
Cottage cheese is high in protein and calcium, which promotes muscle and bone development.
 Lean Proteins: Chicken and turkey are good sources of lean protein. They are high in nutrients like as iron, which is essential for red blood cell synthesis.
Fish: Certain fish species, such as salmon, trout, and sardines, are high in omega-3 fatty acids, which are essential for newborn brain and eye development. Pregnant women should be vigilant about mercury levels in fish and avoid high-mercury seafood such as swordfish and shark.

Lean Beef: Lean cuts of beef include high-quality protein, iron, and B vitamins, all of which are vital for the health of both the mother and the infant.

Legumes, such as beans, lentils, and chickpeas, are high in protein, fibre, iron, and folate, all of which are essential for preventing birth abnormalities.

Whole grains:

1.Quinoa: It is a complete protein, supplying all essential amino acids, along with fiber and iron, magnesium and B-vitamins.

Brown rice is a healthier alternative to white rice since it contains more fiber, B vitamins, and minerals such as selenium and magnesium.

2.Oats: Oats are high in fiber and include a variety of critical minerals such as iron, B vitamins, and antioxidants, which promote digestive health.

Whole wheat products, such as bread, pasta, and couscous, are rich in fiber, B vitamins, and minerals like selenium and magnesium.

Pregnant women should eat a well-balanced diet rich in fruits, vegetables, and dairy products to ensure they acquire enough nutrients for their own health and the development of their baby. However, it is recommended that you speak with a healthcare expert or a nutritionist to personalize dietary advice based on your specific needs and health problems while pregnant.

3.Stay Hydrated: Drink enough water to stay properly hydrated.

4.Exercise: Perform prenatal exercises recommended by your healthcare physician. Walking, swimming, and yoga can all help you feel better and stay fit.

5.Adequate Rest: Get enough sleep and take naps as needed. Pregnancy can be physically demanding, so relaxation is essential.

Emotional well-being:

Pregnancy affects both the mother and the baby's emotional well-being. It includes a woman's mental and emotional state throughout her pregnancy, which affects her overall health and the prenatal environment. Here are the important aspects:

1.Mental Health: Pregnancy can cause a wide range of feelings, from happiness and enthusiasm to anxiety and stress. Hormonal changes, physical discomfort, and the expectation of childbirth can all have an impact on a woman's mental health. Conditions like depression, anxiety, and mood disorders can emerge or worsen during this time, necessitating prompt attention and support.

2.Stress Management: High levels of stress can have an influence on both the mother's health and the baby's growth. Mindfulness, meditation, yoga, and deep breathing exercises can all help reduce stress and increase relaxation.

3.Body Image and Self-Esteem: Physical changes that occur during pregnancy can have an impact on a woman's body image and self-esteem. Accepting these changes and keeping a positive body image are critical for emotional health.
4.Communication: Share any concerns or fears with your partner, healthcare provider, or counselor. Open conversation can reduce anxiety and provide a sense of reassurance.

Comfort

1.Comfortable Clothing: Invest in comfortable pregnancy clothing that fits your developing body. Supportive bras, loose-fitting clothing, and pregnancy belts can provide comfort.

2.Rest and Relaxation: Take warm baths, utilize pregnancy pillows for support while sleeping, and stretch gently to relieve discomfort.
3.Toxin Avoidance: Avoid alcohol, smoking, and exposure to chemicals that can impair the baby's development.

Education and preparation:

1.Prenatal Classes: Attending prenatal classes will help you learn about birthing, breastfeeding, and baby care. This information can increase confidence and reduce anxiety.
2.Birth Plan: Talk to your healthcare provider about your birth preferences and develop a flexible birth plan that fits your needs.

Choices of giving birth

The water birth procedure: for a water birth, it is giving birth in a warm water tub.
Benefits: Offers buoyancy, relieving pressure on the body; may ease pain and induce relaxation.
Limitations in some medical circumstances; meticulous water temperature monitoring and infection control are necessary.
Setting: May take place at clinics, hospitals, or, in rare occasions, at home with medical support.

Process of a Normal Labour Birth (virginal birth):
Natural birth via the birth canal.
Advantages: Generally less time spent recovering; helps strengthen the mother-child attachment.
Taking into account: The possibility of suffering and the potential need for medical measures.

Setting: Depending on the person's health and choices, this can happen at home, at a hospital, or at a birthing center.

Cesarean section(C-section): Procedure: An abdominal and uterine incision is made during surgery to deliver the baby.
Advantages: Essential in particular medical situations or emergencies; sometimes prearranged.

Compared to vaginal birth, there is a longer recovery period and a higher chance of complications.
Setting: Usually in hospitals; may be scheduled or carried out on short notice.
Every birthing choice offers benefits and things to keep in mind of its own. To make an informed selection, it's crucial to speak with healthcare specialists about a person's preferences, medical issues, and overall health.

3.Prepare Your Home: Gather baby supplies, set up the nursery, and make plans for post-birth care.
Monitoring and Self-Care:
1.Monitor Symptoms: Be alert and report any unexpected symptoms or changes to your healthcare professional right once.
2.Self-care Rituals: Do things that encourage relaxation and happiness, such reading, listening to music, or pursuing hobbies.

Conclusion

Enjoying parenthood after a pregnancy is a complex process that extends beyond the initial stages of bringing a new life into the world. It entails fostering bonds between people, respecting both unique and shared experiences, and laying the groundwork for a strong and happy family life.Be it recognising the difficulties or embracing cultural customs, building a network of support or strengthening sibling relationships, the joy of parenthood is an ongoing adventure filled with development, education, and making treasured memories. It involves writing a family history that captures the ideals, goals, and distinct personalities of each individual.It becomes crucial for parents to modify traditions for contemporary families and include mindful parenting techniques as they negotiate the challenges of raising a child. The family's future vision, milestones that are celebrated together, and daily routines are all part of the celebration.In the end, the celebration of parenthood is a continuous dedication to love, care, and develop as a family. It's a never-ending tale of resiliency, happiness, and the unbreakable relationship that turns two people into devoted parents and sets off a journey that alters the trajectory of a lifetime.

Fertility, conception, and pregnancy are all significant stages in the human life cycle.These interwoven stages represent the various biological processes and emotional experiences that comprise the wonder of birth.Fertility, the basis of this journey, represents the delicate balance of many factors;hormonal, environmental, and genetic, that influence a person's capacity to conceive. It's a complicated interplay in which health, lifestyle decisions, and medical interventions frequently intersect, influencing the likelihood of successful conception. Conception, or the merging of egg and sperm, signifies the beginning of new life. It captures the awe-inspiring moment when cells begin to divide and create the foundation of a distinct human person.This point serves as a tribute to both the amazing journey that lies ahead and the marvels of biology.

The changing phase of pregnancy includes a wide range of physiological, psychological, and emotional changes. The first few weeks are a time of great significance and expectation, as they are dedicated to the development of a fetus's key organs and its amazing growth. The pregnant person experiences a remarkable journey, appreciating the amazing process of nourishing life while navigating several milestones and hurdles.

It is impossible to overestimate the importance of complete healthcare, emotional support, and well-informed decision-making during these phases. Every stage has its own pleasures, challenges, and obligations, which emphasizes how crucial it is to have access to high-quality medical care, education, and support systems.

To sum up, conception, pregnancy, and fertility capture the wonders of life, the intricacies of biology, and the deep process of bringing a new life into the world, and they represent the core of the human experience. It is evidence of the human body's tenacity, wonder, and beauty as well as the depths of the human spirit's emotions.

9 798887 338899